It's easy to get lost in the cancer world

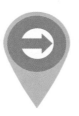

Let
**NCCN Guidelines
for Patients®
be your guide**

✓ Step-by-step guides to the cancer care options likely to have the best results

✓ Based on treatment guidelines used by health care providers worldwide

✓ Designed to help you discuss cancer treatment with your doctors

T0204582

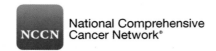

National Comprehensive
Cancer Network®

NCCN Guidelines for Patients® are developed by the National Comprehensive Cancer Network® (NCCN®)

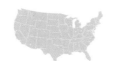

NCCN

✓ An alliance of leading cancer centers across the United States devoted to patient care, research, and education

Cancer centers that are part of NCCN:
NCCN.org/cancercenters

NCCN Clinical Practice Guidelines in Oncology (NCCN Guidelines®)

✓ Developed by experts from NCCN cancer centers using the latest research and years of experience

✓ For providers of cancer care all over the world

✓ Expert recommendations for cancer screening, diagnosis, and treatment

Free online at
NCCN.org/guidelines

NCCN Guidelines for Patients

✓ Present information from the NCCN Guidelines in an easy-to-learn format

✓ For people with cancer and those who support them

✓ Explain the cancer care options likely to have the best results

Free online at
NCCN.org/patientguidelines

These NCCN Guidelines for Patients are based on the NCCN Guidelines® for Breast Cancer, Version 2.2022 – December 20, 2021.

NCCN Foundation seeks to support the millions of patients and their families affected by a cancer diagnosis by funding and distributing NCCN Guidelines for Patients. NCCN Foundation is also committed to advancing cancer treatment by funding the nation's promising doctors at the center of innovation in cancer research. For more details and the full library of patient and caregiver resources, visit NCCN.org/patients.

National Comprehensive Cancer Network (NCCN) / NCCN Foundation
3025 Chemical Road, Suite 100
Plymouth Meeting, PA 19462
215.690.0300

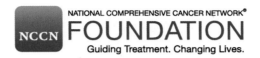

NATIONAL COMPREHENSIVE CANCER NETWORK®
FOUNDATION
Guiding Treatment. Changing Lives.

NCCN Guidelines for Patients are supported by funding from the NCCN Foundation®

To make a gift or learn more, please visit NCCNFoundation.org/donate
or e-mail PatientGuidelines@NCCN.org.

Brem Foundation

The Brem Foundation teaches women about the need for personalized screening, opens access to breast care for women in need, and advocates for public policies that increase women's opportunities to screen for breast cancer. The Brem Foundation prides itself on reaching women from all socio-economic backgrounds and has made social determinants of health a large focus in all of its work. bremfoundation.org

With additional support from Dr. Wui-Jin Koh

In honor of Judy Anne Hanada Koh

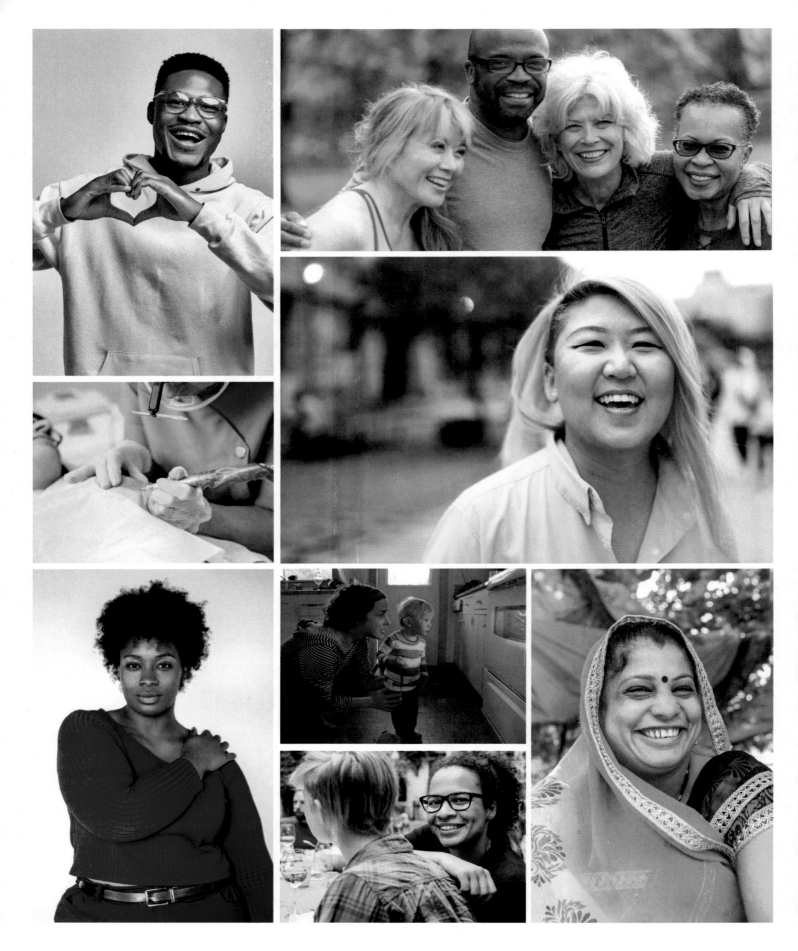

Contents

1

Breast cancer basics

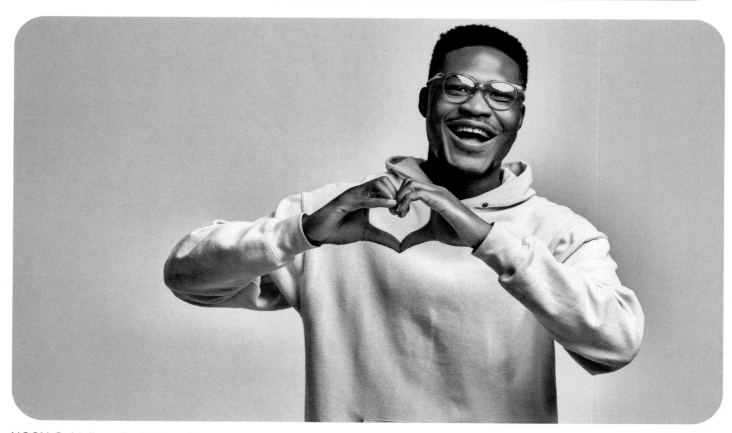

Ductal carcinoma in situ (DCIS) is a type of cancer of the cells that line the ducts found in the breast. DCIS is stage 0 or noninvasive cancer. This means the cancerous cells are in place (in situ) and have not spread outside the ducts. DCIS is treated to prevent invasive breast cancer, a more serious form of cancer.

The breast

The breast is an organ and a gland found on the chest. The breast is made of milk ducts, fat, nerves, lymph and blood vessels, ligaments, and other connective tissue. Behind the breast is the pectoral (chest) muscle and ribs. Muscle and ligaments help hold the breast in place.

Breast tissue contains glands that can make milk. These milk glands are called lobules. Lobules look like tiny clusters of grapes. Small tubes called ducts connect the lobules to the nipple.

The ring of darker breast skin is called the areola. The raised tip within the areola is called the nipple. The nipple-areola complex (NAC) is a term that refers to both parts.

Lymph is a clear fluid that gives cells water and food. It also helps to fight germs. Lymph drains from breast tissue into lymph vessels and travels to lymph nodes near your armpit (axilla). Nodes near the armpit are called axillary lymph nodes (ALNs).

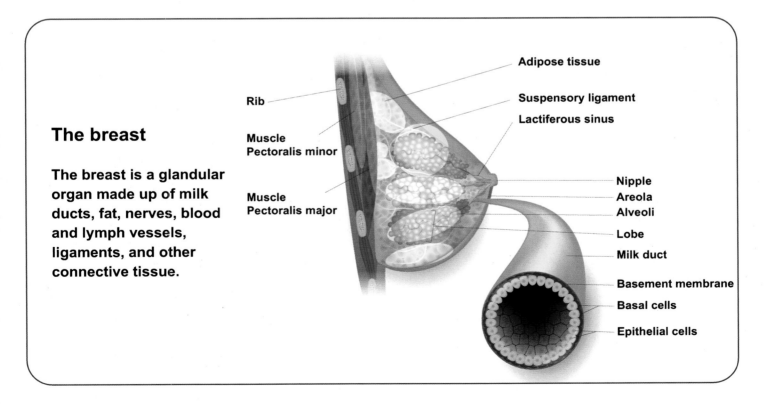

The breast

The breast is a glandular organ made up of milk ducts, fat, nerves, blood and lymph vessels, ligaments, and other connective tissue.

Rib

Muscle Pectoralis minor

Muscle Pectoralis major

Adipose tissue

Suspensory ligament

Lactiferous sinus

Nipple

Areola

Alveoli

Lobe

Milk duct

Basement membrane

Basal cells

Epithelial cells

Ductal carcinoma in situ

Ductal carcinoma in situ (DCIS) is a type of cancer of the cells that line the ducts. Ducts are thin tubes that carry milk in the breast. DCIS is noninvasive. Noninvasive means the cancerous cells are in place (in situ) and have not spread. Anyone can deveop this kind of breast cancer, including males. Ductal carcinoma in situ is also called intraductal carcinoma. You may hear that DCIS is pre-invasive or pre-cancerous. DCIS is treated to prevent invasive breast cancer, a more advanced form of cancer.

Lobular carcinoma in situ

Lobular carcinoma in situ (LCIS) is a benign (non-cancerous) condition in which abnormal cells are found in the lobules of the breast. Having LCIS in one breast increases the risk of developing breast cancer in either breast. LCIS is not covered in this book.

How breast cancer spreads

Cancer cells don't behave like normal cells. Cancer cells differ from normal cells in the following ways.

Primary tumor

Over time, cancer cells form a mass called a primary tumor.

Invasive

Cancer cells can grow into surrounding tissues. Invasive breast cancer is breast cancer that has spread from the milk ducts or milk glands (lobules) into the surrounding breast tissue or nearby lymph nodes.

For more information on invasive breast cancer, read the *NCCN Guidelines for Patients®: Breast Cancer – Invasive*, available at NCCN.org/patientguidelines.

Metastasis

Unlike normal cells, cancer cells can spread and form tumors in other parts of the body. Cancer that has spread is called a metastasis. In this process, cancer cells break away from the first (primary) tumor and travel through blood or lymph vessels to distant sites. Once in other sites, cancer cells may form secondary tumors.

For more information on metastatic breast cancer, read the *NCCN Guidelines for Patients®: Breast Cancer – Metastatic* available at NCCN.org/patientguidelines.

Key points

- Anyone can develop breast cancer.

- Inside breasts are lobules, ducts, fat, blood and lymph vessels, ligaments, and connective tissue. Lobules are structures that make breast milk. Ducts carry breast milk from the lobules to the nipple.

- Breast cancer often starts in the ducts or lobules and then spreads into the surrounding tissue.

- Breast cancer that is found only inside the ducts or lobules is called noninvasive. Ductal carcinoma in situ (DCIS) is found only in the ducts.

- Invasive breast cancer is cancer that has grown outside the ducts or lobules into surrounding tissue. Once outside the ducts or lobules, breast cancer can spread through lymph or blood to lymph nodes or other parts of the body.

- Metastatic breast cancer has spread to distant sites in the body.

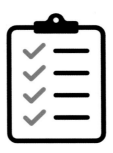

We want your feedback!

Our goal is to provide helpful and easy-to-understand information on cancer.

Take our survey to let us know what we got right and what we could do better:

NCCN.org/patients/feedback

2
Testing for DCIS

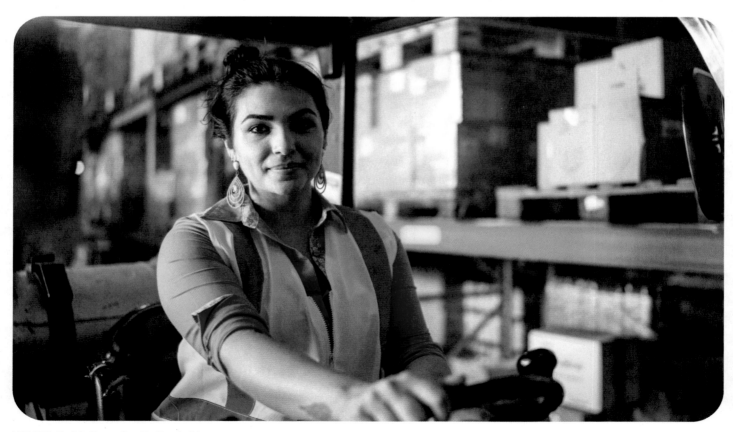

Treatment planning starts with testing. This chapter presents an overview of the tests you might receive and what to expect.

Test results

Results from imaging studies and biopsy will be used to determine your treatment plan. It is important you understand what these tests mean. Ask questions and keep copies of your test results. Online patient portals are a great way to access your test results.

Keep these things in mind:

> Bring someone with you to doctor visits, if possible.

> Write down questions and take notes during appointments. Don't be afraid to ask your care team questions. Get to know your care team and help them get to know you.

> Get copies of blood tests, imaging results, and reports about the specific type of cancer you have.

> Organize your papers. Create files for insurance forms, medical records, and test results. You can do the same on your computer.

> Keep a list of contact information for everyone on your care team. Add it to your phone. Hang the list on your refrigerator or keep it in a place where someone can access it in an emergency. Keep your primary care physician informed of changes to this list.

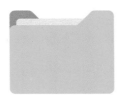

Create a medical binder

A medical binder or notebook is a great way to organize all of your records in one place.

• Make copies of blood tests, imaging results, and reports about your specific type of cancer. It will be helpful when getting a second opinion.

• Choose a binder that meets your needs. Consider a zipper pocket to include a pen, small calendar, and insurance cards.

• Create folders for insurance forms, medical records, and tests results. You can do the same on your computer.

• Use online patient portals to view your test results and other records. Download or print the records to add to your binder.

• Organize your binder in a way that works for you. Add a section for questions and to take notes.

• Bring your medical binder to appointments. You never know when you might need it!

General health tests

Medical history

A medical history is a record of all health issues and treatments you have had in your life. Be prepared to list any illness or injury and when it happened. Bring a list of old and new medicines and any over-the-counter medicines, herbals, or supplements you take. Tell your doctor about any symptoms you have. A medical history, sometimes called a health history, will help determine which treatment is best for you.

Family history

Some cancers and other diseases can run in families. Your doctor will ask about the health history of family members who are blood relatives. This information is called a family history. You can ask family members about their health issues like heart disease, cancer, and diabetes, and at what age they were diagnosed.

Physical exam

During a physical exam, your health care provider may:

> Check your temperature, blood pressure, pulse, and breathing rate

> Check your weight and height

> Listen to your lungs and heart

> Look in your eyes, ears, nose, and throat

> Feel and apply pressure to parts of your body to see if organs are of normal size, are soft or hard, or cause pain when touched. Tell your doctor if you feel pain.

> Examine your breasts to look for lumps, nipple discharge or bleeding, or skin changes. Tell your doctor if you have noticed changes in your breast(s).

> Feel for enlarged lymph nodes in your neck and underarm. Tell your doctor if you have felt any lumps or have any pain.

For possible tests, see Guide 1.

Guide 1 Possible tests
Medical history and physical exam
Diagnostic bilateral mammogram
Pathology review
Determine estrogen receptor (ER) status
Genetic counseling if at risk for hereditary breast cancer
Breast MRI, as needed

Fertility

Treatment can affect your fertility, the ability to have children. If you think you want children in the future, ask your doctor how cancer and cancer treatment might change your fertility. In order to preserve your fertility, you may need to take action before starting cancer treatment. Those who want to have children in the future should be referred to a fertility specialist to discuss the options before starting treatment.

Fertility preservation is all about keeping your options open, whether you know you want to have children later in life or aren't really sure at the moment. Fertility and reproductive specialists can help you sort through what may be best for your situation.

More information on fertility preservation can be found in the *NCCN Guidelines for Patients®: Adolescents and Young Adults with Cancer*, available at NCCN.org/patientguidelines.

Impaired fertility
Treatment for DCIS might cause your fertility to be temporarily impaired or interrupted. This temporary loss of fertility is related to your age at time of diagnosis, treatment type(s), treatment dose, and treatment length. Talk to your doctor about your concerns and if you are planning a pregnancy.

Preventing pregnancy

Preventing pregnancy during treatment is important. Cancer and cancer treatment can affect the ovaries and damage sperm. Hormonal birth control may not be recommended, so ask your doctor about options such as intrauterine devices (IUDs) and barrier methods. Types of barrier methods include condoms, diaphragms, cervical caps, and the contraceptive sponge.

Those with ovaries
Those who can become pregnant will have a pregnancy test before starting treatment. Cancer treatment can hurt the baby if you are or become pregnant during treatment. Therefore, birth control to prevent pregnancy during and after treatment is recommended. Also, consult your doctor for the best time to plan a pregnancy.

Those with testicles
Cancer and cancer treatment can damage sperm. Therefore, use contraception (birth control) such as condoms to prevent pregnancy during and after cancer treatment. If you think you want children in the future, talk to your doctor now. Sperm banking is an option.

Menstruation
Menstruation, menses, menstrual flow, or your "period" may stop during treatment, but often returns within 2 years after treatment in those 40 years of age and under.It is still possible to become pregnant even though you might not have a period. Therefore, birth control is recommended during and after treatment.

Treatment during pregnancy
Certain treatments will need to be avoided if you are pregnant or breastfeeding.

Imaging tests

Imaging tests take pictures of the inside of your body. These tests are used to find and treat DCIS. Imaging tests show the primary tumor, or where the cancer started, and look for cancer in other parts of the body. A radiologist, an expert in interpreting imaging tests, will write a report and send this report to your doctor. Your doctor will discuss the results with you.

Diagnostic bilateral mammogram
A mammogram is a picture of the inside of your breast. The picture is made using x-rays. A computer combines the x-rays to make detailed pictures. Mammogram results are used to plan treatment.

Diagnostic mammograms look at specific areas of your breasts, which may not be clearly seen on screening mammograms. It is used to see tumor and the size of the tumor(s). Other tests may include a breast MRI or ultrasound.

Breast MRI
A magnetic resonance imaging (MRI) scan uses radio waves and powerful magnets to take pictures of the inside of the body. It does not use x-rays. If needed, an MRI would be used in addition to a mammogram. Tell your doctor if you have any metal in your body.

In most cases, contrast will be used. Contrast material is used to improve the pictures of the inside of the body. Contrast materials are not dyes, but substances that help enhance and improve the images of several organs and structures in the body. It is used to make the pictures clearer. The contrast is not

> Imaging and other tests are not always accurate. A multidisciplinary team should review the results.

permanent and will leave the body in your urine immediately after the test.

Tell your doctors if you have had allergic reactions to contrast in the past. This is important. You might be given medicines, such as Benadryl and prednisone, to avoid the effects of those allergies. Contrast might not be used if you have a serious allergy or if your kidneys aren't working well.

Ultrasound
An ultrasound (US) uses high-energy sound waves to form pictures of the inside of the body. This is similar to the sonogram used for pregnancy. Ultrasound is painless and does not use x-rays, so it can be repeated as needed. Ultrasound is good at showing small areas of cancer that are near the skin. Sometimes, a breast ultrasound or MRI is used to guide a biopsy.

Biopsy

A biopsy is a procedure that removes a sample of tissue or fluid. The sample is sent to a lab for testing. A pathologist will examine the biopsy for cancer and write a report called a pathology report. Ask questions about your biopsy results and what it means for your treatment.

There are different types of biopsies. Some biopsies are guided using imaging, such as mammmogram, ultrasound, or MRI. The primary or main tumor is biopsied first. Other tumors or tumors in different areas may also be biopsied. You may have tissue removed from the breast, lymph nodes, or both.

Types of possible biopsies include:

> **Fine-needle aspiration (FNA) or core biopsy (CB)** uses needles of different sizes to remove a sample of tissue or fluid.

> **Excisional biopsy** removes a small amount of tissue through a cut in the skin or body.

Sentinel lymph node biopsy

A sentinel lymph node (SLN) is the first lymph node that cancer cells are most likely to spread to from a primary tumor. Often, there is more than one sentinel lymph node. Removal of the sentinel lymph nodes during surgery is called a sentinel lymph node biopsy (SLNB or SNB). This procedure is done during surgery such as a mastectomy (surgery to remove the breast) or lumpectomy (surgery to remove the tumor) to determine if any cancer cells have

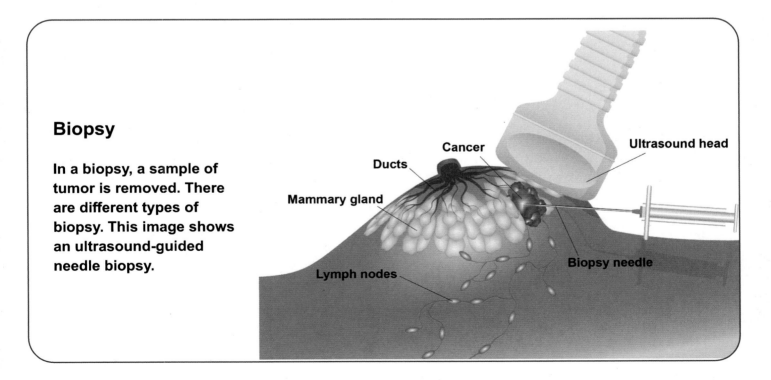

Biopsy

In a biopsy, a sample of tumor is removed. There are different types of biopsy. This image shows an ultrasound-guided needle biopsy.

traveled to the lymph nodes. The lymph nodes removed are called the sentinel nodes. They may or may not contain any cancer cells. Just because these nodes are removed, it does not mean that they are positive for cancer.

To find the sentinel lymph nodes, a radioactive material and other dyes are injected into the body near the breast where they travel through the lymphatics in the breast to the lymph nodes. This helps the surgeon find which of the nodes are the sentinel lymph nodes. Once the nodes are found, those containing the radioactive materal or dye are removed and tested by a pathologist. If cancer is found, then more than one lymph node may be removed.

Estrogen receptor status

Estrogen is a hormone that plays a role in breast development. A hormone is a substance made by a gland in your body. Your blood carries hormones throughout your body. A receptor is a protein found inside or on the surface of a cell. Substances such as hormones attach (bind) to these receptors. This causes changes within the cell.

Hormones recognize and bind to specific hormone receptors. When hormones, such as estrogen, attach to receptors inside breast cancer cells, they can cause cancer to grow. If found, these estrogen receptors may be targeted for treatment using endocrine therapy.

Immunohistochemistry
Immunohistochemistry (IHC) is a special staining process that involves adding a chemical marker to cells. These cells are then studied using a microscope. IHC can find estrogen receptors in breast cancer cells. A pathologist will measure how many cells have estrogen receptors and the number of estrogen receptors inside each cell. Test results will either be estrogen receptor-positive (ER+) or estrogen receptor-negative (ER-).

Estrogen receptor-positive
In estrogen receptor-positive (ER+) breast cancer, IHC finds estrogen hormone receptors in at least 1 out of every 100 cancer cells. ER+ cancer cells may need estrogen to grow. These cells may stop growing or die with treatment to block estrogen called endocrine therapy.

Estrogen receptor-negative
Estrogen receptor-negative (ER-) breast cancer cells do not have estrogen hormone receptors. These cancer cells do not need estrogen to grow and continue to grow despite treatment to block estrogen.

HER2 status

Human epidermal growth factor receptor 2 (HER2) is a protein involved in normal cell growth. It is found on the surface of all cells. HER2 testing is not done for DCIS. HER2 status does not affect treatment options for DCIS. HER2 testing is done for invasive and metastatic breast cancer.

Genetic risk testing

About 1 out of 10 breast cancers are hereditary. Depending on your family history or other features of your cancer, your health care provider might refer you for hereditary genetic testing to learn more about your cancer. A genetic counselor or trained provider will speak to you about the results. Tests results may be used to guide treatment planning.

Genetic testing is done using blood or saliva (spitting into a cup). The goal is to look for gene mutations inherited from your biological parents called germline mutations. Some mutations can put you at risk for more than one type of cancer. You can pass these genes on to your children. Also, family members might carry these mutations. Tell your doctor if there is a family history of cancer.

BRCA tests

Everyone has *BRCA* genes. Normal *BRCA* genes help to prevent tumor growth. They help fix damaged cells and help cells grow normally. *BRCA* mutations put you at risk for more than one type of cancer. Mutations in *BRCA1* or *BRCA2* increase the risk of breast, ovarian, prostate, colorectal, pancreatic, and melanoma skin cancers. Mutated *BRCA* genes can also affect how well some treatments work. These tests might be repeated.

What is your family health history?

Some cancers and other diseases run in families – those who are related to you – through genes passed down from parent to child. This information is called a family health history. You can ask family members about their health issues like heart disease, cancer, and diabetes, and at what age they were diagnosed. For relatives who have died, ask about the cause and age of death.

Start by asking your parents, siblings, and children. Next, talk to half-siblings, aunts and uncles, niece and nephews, grandparents, and grandchildren.

Write down what you learn about your family history and share with your health care provider.

Some of the questions to ask include:

- Do you have any chronic diseases, such as heart disease or diabetes, or health conditions such as high blood pressure or high cholesterol?

- Have you had any other diseases, such as cancer or stroke?

- How old were you when each of these diseases and health conditions was diagnosed?

- What is our family's ancestry – from what countries did our ancestors originate?

Cancer stages

Breast cancer staging is often done twice.

> **Clinical stage (c)** is the rating given before any treatment. It is based on a physical exam, biopsy, and imaging tests. An example might look like cT0 or cN1.

> **Pathologic stage (p)** or surgical stage is determined by examining tissue removed during surgery. An example might be pT1.

A cancer stage is a way to describe the extent of the cancer at the time you are first diagnosed. The American Joint Committee on Cancer (AJCC) created a staging system to determine how much cancer is in your body, where it is located, and what subtype you have. AJCC is just one type of staging system.

Staging is based on a combination of information to reach a final numbered stage. Often, not all information is available at the initial evaluation. More information can be gathered as treatment begins. Doctors may explain your cancer stage in different ways than described next.

TNM scores

The tumor, node, metastasis (TNM) system is used to stage breast cancer. In this system, the letters T, N, and M describe different areas of cancer growth. Based on cancer test results, your doctor will assign a score or number to each letter. The higher the number, the larger the tumor or the more the cancer has spread. These scores will be combined to assign the cancer a stage. A TNM example might look like this: T1N0M0 or T1, N0, M0, or for DCIS TisN0M0.

> **T (tumor)** – Depth and spread of the main (primary) tumor(s) in one or both breasts

> **N (node)** - If cancer has spread to nearby (regional) lymph nodes

> **M (metastasis)** - If cancer has spread to distant parts of the body or metastasized

Lymph nodes

Lymph, a clear fluid containing cells that help fight infections and other diseases, drains through channels into lymphatic vessels. From here, lymph drains into lymph nodes. Lymph nodes work as filters to help fight infection and remove harmful things from your body. Regional lymph nodes are found near the breast. It is possible for cancerous cells to travel through lymph to other parts of the body.

Grade

Grade describes how abnormal the tumor cells look under a microscope (called histology). Higher-grade cancers tend to grow and spread faster than lower-grade cancers. GX means the grade can't be determined, followed by G1, G2, and G3. G3 is the highest grade for breast cancers. A low-grade tumor has a low risk of recurrence. A high-grade tumor has a higher risk for recurrence (of cancer returning)

> **GX** – Grade cannot be determined

> **G1** – Low (nuclear grade 1)

> **G2** – Intermediate (nuclear grade 2)

> **G3** – High (nuclear grade 3)

Numbered stages

Numbered stages are based on TNM scores. Stages range from stage 0 to stage 4, with 4 being the most advanced. Doctors write these stages as stage 0, stage I, stage II, stage III, and stage IV. For example, DCIS is stage 0 or Tis, N0, M0.

Stage 0 is noninvasive

Noninvasive breast cancer is rated stage 0. DCIS is found only in the ducts (Tis). It has not spread to the surrounding breast tissue, lymph nodes (N0) or distant sites (M0).

Stages 1, 2, and 3 are invasive

Invasive breast cancer is rated stage 1, 2, or 3. It has grown outside the ducts, lobules, or breast skin. Cancer might be in the axillary lymph nodes.

For more information on invasive breast cancer, read the *NCCN Guidelines for Patients®: Breast Cancer – Invasive*, available at NCCN.org/patientguidelines.

Stage 4 is metastatic

In stage 4 breast cancer, cancer has spread to distant sites. It can develop from earlier stages. Rarely, your first diagnosis can be stage 4 metastatic breast cancer (called de novo) or it can develop from earlier stages.

For more information on metastatic breast cancer, read the *NCCN Guidelines for Patients®: Breast Cancer – Metastatic* available at NCCN.org/patientguidelines.

Breast sections

Quadrants are used to describe tumor location. Each breast is divided into 4 sections or quadrants. They are the upper outer quadrant (near the armpit), the upper inner quadrant (near the center of the body), the lower outer quadrant, and the lower inner quadrant. The nipple area is called the nipple-areola complex (NAC).

https://commons.wikimedia.org/wiki/File:Breast_quadrants.svg

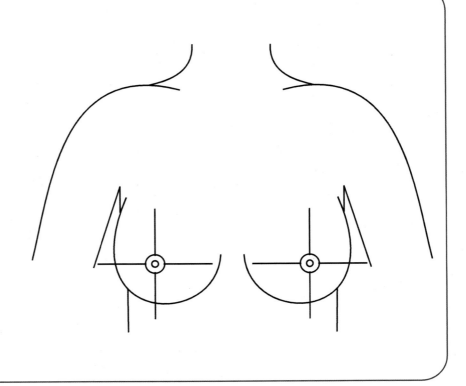

Key points

> Tests are used to find cancer, plan treatment, and check how well treatment is working.

> You will have a physical exam, including a breast exam, to see if anything feels or looks abnormal.

> Treatment can affect your fertility, the ability to have children.

> Imaging tests take pictures of the inside of your body.

> A diagnostic bilateral mammogram includes detailed pictures of both breasts. It is different than a screening mammogram.

> During a biopsy, tissue or fluid samples are removed for testing.

> A sample from a biopsy of your tumor will be tested for estrogen receptor (ER) status and grade (histology).

> Some breast cancers grow because of estrogen. Testing will be done to see if you have estrogen receptor-positive (ER+) breast cancer.

> About 1 out of 10 breast cancers are hereditary. Depending on your family history or other features of your cancer, your health care provider might refer you for hereditary genetic testing or to speak with a genetic counselor.

> A cancer stage is a way to describe the extent of the cancer at the time you are first diagnosed.

> Breast cancer is often staged twice, before and after surgery.

> A sentinel lymph node (SLN) is the first lymph node(s) that cancer cells are most likely to spread to from a primary tumor. A sentinel lymph node biopsy (SNLB) might be done to look for cancer in your lymph node(s).

> Online portals are a great way to access your test results.

HER2 testing is not used in the diagnosis and treatment of DCIS.

3
Treatment overview

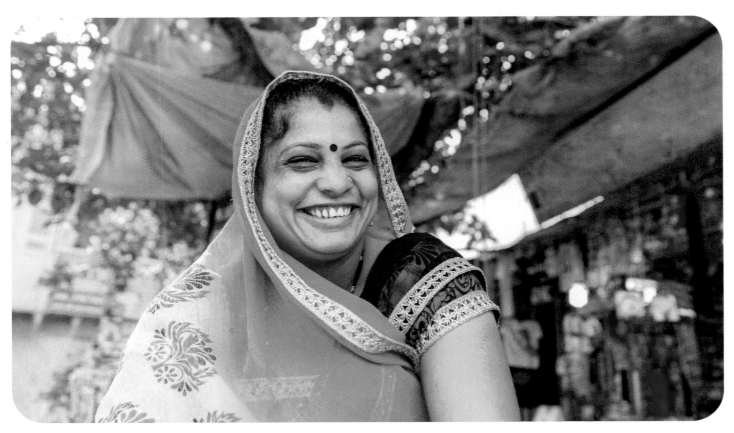

There is more than one treatment for DCIS. This chapter describes treatment options and what to expect. Together, you and your doctor will choose a treatment plan that is best for you.

Treatment team

Treating breast cancer takes a team approach. Treatment decisions should involve a multidisciplinary team (MDT). An MDT is a team of doctors, health care workers, and social care professionals from different professional backgrounds who have knowledge (expertise) and experience with your type of cancer. This team is united in the planning and implementing of your treatment. Ask who will coordinate your care.

Some members of your care team will be with you throughout cancer treatment, while others will only be there for parts of it. Get to know your care team and help them get to know you.

Depending on your diagnosis, your team might include the following:

> **A pathologist** analyzes the cells, tissues, and organs removed during a biopsy or surgery and provides cancer diagnosis, staging, and information about biomarker testing.

> **A diagnostic radiologist** interprets the results of x-rays and other imaging tests.

> **A surgical oncologist** performs operations to remove cancer.

> **A reconstructive (plastic) surgeon** performs breast reconstruction, if desired, for those who undergo mastectomy.

> **A medical oncologist** treats cancer in adults using systemic (drug) therapy.

> **A radiation oncologist** prescribes and plans radiation therapy to treat cancer.

> **An anesthesiologist** gives anesthesia, a medicine so you do not feel pain during surgery or procedures.

> **Residents and fellows** are doctors who are continuing their training, some to become specialists in a certain field of medicine.

> **Nurse practitioners and physician assistants** are health care providers who work alongside doctors and other members of the medical team. Some of your clinic visits may be done by a nurse practitioner or physician assistant.

> **Oncology nurses** provide your hands-on care, like giving systemic therapy, managing your care, answering questions, and helping you cope with side effects. Sometimes, these experts are called nurse navigators.

> **Oncology pharmacists** provide medicines used to treat cancer and to manage symptoms and side effects.

> **Nutritionists and dietitians** can provide guidance on what foods are most suitable for your condition.

> **An occupational therapist** helps people with the tasks of daily living.

> **A physical therapist** helps people move with greater comfort and ease.

> **A certified lymphedema therapist** gives a type of massage called manual lymph drainage.

> **Psychologists and psychiatrists** are mental health experts who can help manage issues such as depression, anxiety, or other mental health conditions that can affect how you feel.

> **Social workers** help people solve and cope with problems in their everyday lives. Clinical social workers also diagnose and treat mental, behavioral, and emotional issues. The anxiety a person feels when diagnosed with cancer might well be managed by a social worker in some cancer centers.

> **A research team** helps to collect research data and coordinate care if you are in a clinical trial.

Your physical, mental, and emotional well-being are important. You know yourself better than anyone. Help other team members understand:

> How you feel

> What you need

> What is working and what is not

Keep a list of names and contact information for each member of your team. This will make it easier for you and anyone involved in your care to know whom to contact with questions or concerns.

Get to know your care team and help them get to know you.

Surgery

Surgery is an operation or procedure to remove cancer from the body. Surgery is the main or primary treatment for DCIS. This is only one part of a treatment plan.

When preparing for surgery, seek the opinion of an experienced surgeon. The surgeon should be an expert in performing your type of surgery. Hospitals that perform many surgeries often have better results. You can ask for a referral to a hospital or cancer center that has experience in treating your type of cancer.

The removal of the cancer through surgery can be accomplished in different ways depending on the specific circumstances, such as the size and location of the tumor, and if there is cancer in any surrounding organs and tissues.

Surgery might be a lumpectomy or mastectomy. It is based on the safest and best way to remove the cancer. If you are considering breast reconstruction, surgery requires collaboration between a breast surgeon and a reconstructive (plastic) surgeon. Radiation therapy usually only follows after a lumpectomy. It is important to note that a lymph node biopsy is not done with a lumpectomy.

Goal of surgery

The goal of surgery or tumor resection is to remove all of the cancer. To do so, the tumor is removed along with a rim of normal-looking tissue around its edge called the surgical margin. The surgical margin may look normal during surgery, but cancerous cells may be found when viewed under a microscope by a pathologist. A clear or negative margin (R0) is when no cancer cells are found in the tissue

If you smoke or vape

If you smoke tobacco or use e-cigarettes, it is very important to quit. Smoking can limit how well cancer treatment works. Smoking greatly increases your chances of having side effects during and after surgery, including breast reconstruction. It also increases your chances of developing other cancers.

Nicotine is the chemical in tobacco that makes you want to keep smoking. Nicotine withdrawal is challenging for most smokers. The stress of having cancer may make it even harder to quit. If you smoke, ask your doctor about counseling and medicines to help you quit.

For online support, try these websites:

- SmokeFree.gov
- BeTobaccoFree.gov
- CDC.gov/tobacco

around the edge of the tumor. In a positive margin, cancer cells are found in normal-looking tissue around the tumor.

Surgical margins

The goal of surgery is a cancer-free surgical margin. After surgery, you may receive treatment such as radiation to kill any remaining cancer cells.

> **In a clear or negative margin (R0),** no cancerous cells are found in the tissue around the edge of the tumor.

> **In an R1 positive margin,** the surgeon removes all the visible tumor, but the microscopic margins are still positive for tumor cells. Despite best efforts this can happen.

> **In an R2 positive margin,** the surgeon is unable to remove all the visible tumor or there is metastatic disease.

A negative margin (R0) is the best result. Your surgeon will look carefully for cancer not only along the surgical margin, but in other nearby areas.

Despite best efforts, it is not always possible to find all of the cancer. Sometimes, surgeons can't safely remove the tumor with a cancer-free margin.

You might have more than one surgery. You might also have a wound drain to prevent fluid from collecting in the body after surgery. These drains are usually removed a few days after surgery.

Lumpectomy

Lumpectomy is the removal of abnormal cells or tumor. It is also called breast-conserving therapy or breast-conserving surgery (BCS). In a lumpectomy, only the tumor with an area of normal tissue will be removed. The rest of your breast is left alone. Extra tissue is removed around the tumor to create a cancer-free area. This cancer-free area is called a surgical margin. Having a surgical margin will decrease the chance that cancer may return in that area of the breast. You may have more than one surgery to ensure all of the cancer was removed.

A lumpectomy is usually followed by radiation therapy to part of or the whole breast. A boost is extra radiation to the tumor area.

The breast might not look the same after a lumpectomy. Speak to your doctor about how a lumpectomy might affect the look and shape of your breast, and any concerns you have. Certain reconstruction options, such as volume displacement, might be available.

Breastfeeding

Breastfeeding following a lumpectomy is possible. The quantity and quality of breast milk produced by the breast may not be sufficient or may be lacking some of the nutrients needed. Breastfeeding is not recommended during active treatment or within 6 months of completing certain types of endocrine therapy.

Mastectomy

A mastectomy is surgery to remove all or part of the breast. Lymph nodes and muscle might be removed. Before removing the breast, the surgeon may do a sentinel lymph node biopsy (SLNB). Sentinel lymph nodes are the first lymph nodes cancer cells are likely to have spread from the primary tumor.

Types of mastectomy include:

> **A total mastectomy** or simple mastectomy is a surgery that removes the whole breast with a flat skin closure.

> **A skin-sparing mastectomy** removes the breast but not all of the skin, in order to have breast reconstruction that might include flaps and/or implants.

> **Nipple-sparing mastectomy** preserves the nipple-areola complex (NAC) as well as all of the skin. Not everyone is a candidate for nipple-sparing mastectomy.

Breast reconstruction is an option after a mastectomy. It might be done at the same time as mastectomy ("immediate") or at some time following the completion of cancer treatment ("delayed"). Breast reconstruction is often done in stages.

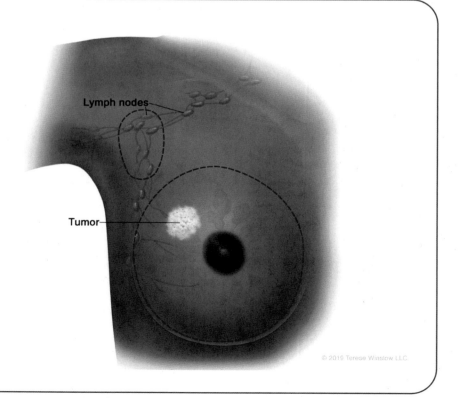

Total simple mastectomy

The dotted line shows where the entire breast is removed. Some lymph nodes under the arm may also be removed.

Lymph nodes

Tumor

© 2019 Terese Winslow LLC

Radiation therapy

Radiation therapy (RT) uses high-energy radiation from x-rays, photons, protons, electrons, and other sources to kill cancer cells and shrink tumors. It is given over a certain period of time. Radiation therapy is given to kill any remaining cancer cells after surgery. Different types of radiation can be used for DCIS. Most types include several short treatment sessions that are given once daily over a few days to weeks. Ask your doctor which radiation option(s) are best for you.

Types of radiation used in DCIS include:

> **Whole breast radiation** is used to treat the entire breast. Sometimes, additional treatments may be given to the tumor area. This is called a "boost."

> **Partial breast radiation** is used to treat only the tumor area of the breast.

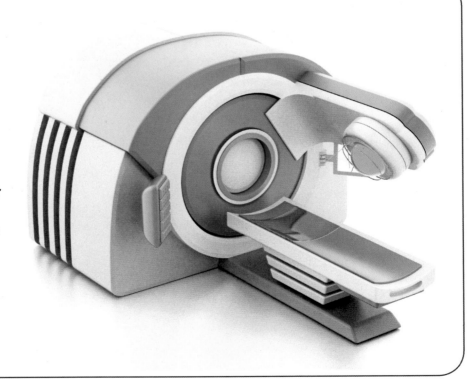

Radiation therapy

Radiation therapy uses high-energy radiation from x-rays, gamma rays, protons, and other sources to kill cancer cells and shrink tumors. It is also used to treat pain caused by cancers.

Endocrine therapy

The endocrine system is made up of organs and tissues that produce hormones. Hormones are natural chemicals released into the bloodstream.

There are 4 hormones that might be targeted in endocrine therapy:

> **Estrogen** is made mainly by the ovaries.

> **Progesterone** is made mainly by the ovaries.

> **Luteinizing hormone-releasing hormone (LHRH)** is made by a part of the brain called the hypothalamus. It tells the ovaries to make estrogen and progesterone and testicles to make testosterone. LHRH is also called gonadotropin-releasing hormone (GnRH).

> **Androgen** is made by the adrenal glands, testicles, and ovaries.

Hormones may cause breast cancer to grow. Endocrine therapy will stop your body from making hormones or it will block what hormones do in the body. This can slow tumor growth or shrink the tumor for a period of time. In DCIS, endocrine therapy is used to reduce the risk of cancer recurrence.

Endocrine therapy is sometimes called hormone therapy. It is not the same as hormone replacement therapy used for menopause.

Types of endocrine therapy that might be used for DCIS:

> **Aromatase inhibitors (AIs)** stop a type of hormone called androgen from changing into estrogen by interfering with an enzyme called aromatase. They do not affect estrogen made by the ovaries. Non-steroidal aromatase inhibitors include anastrozole (Arimidex) and letrozole (Femara). Exemestane (Aromasin) is a steroidal aromatase inhibitor.

> **Estrogen receptor (ER) modulators** or anti-estrogens prevent hormones from binding to receptors.

  · **Selective estrogen receptor modulators (SERMs)** block estrogen from attaching to hormone receptors. They include tamoxifen and toremifene (Fareston).

  · **Selective estrogen receptor degraders (SERDs)** block and destroy estrogen receptors. Fulvestrant (Faslodex) is a SERD.

> **Gonadotropin-releasing hormone (GnRH) agonists** might be used to suppress ovarian hormone or testosterone production.

Those who want to have children in the future should be referred to a fertility specialist before starting endocrine therapy to discuss the options.

Menopausal status

Options for endocrine therapy are partly based on if you started or were in menopause before beginning treatment. In menopause, the ovaries permanently stop producing hormones and menstrual periods stop. After menopause, estrogen and progesterone levels continue to stay low. Cancer treatment can cause a temporary menopause.

Premenopause

If you have menstrual periods, you are in premenopause. In premenopause, the ovaries are the main source of estrogen and progesterone. Menstrual periods may stop during treatment and for up to 2 years after treatment, but often returns in those 40 years of age and under.

Tamoxifen is the endocrine treatment for those in premenopause.

Menopause

When menstrual periods stop for 12 months or more, it is called menopause. If you don't have periods, a test using a blood sample may be needed to confirm your status. In menopause, your adrenal glands, liver, and body fat make small amounts of estrogen.

Tamoxifen or an aromatase inhibitor is the endocrine treatment for those in menopause. Aromatase inhibitors include anastrozole (Arimidex), exemestane (Aromasin), and letrozol (Femara).

> Those who want to have children in the future should be referred to a fertility specialist before starting endocrine therapy.

Testosterone

For those assigned male at birth whose bodies continue to make testosterone, endocrine therapy includes tamoxifen or an aromatase inhibitor with testosterone-suppressing therapy.

Clinical trials

A clinical trial is a type of medical research study. After being developed and tested in a laboratory, potential new ways of fighting cancer need to be studied in people. If found to be safe and effective in a clinical trial, a drug, device, or treatment approach may be approved by the U.S. Food and Drug Administration (FDA).

Everyone with cancer should carefully consider all of the treatment options available for their cancer type, including standard treatments and clinical trials. Talk to your doctor about whether a clinical trial may make sense for you.

Phases

Most cancer clinical trials focus on treatment. Treatment trials are done in phases.

> **Phase I trials** study the dose, safety, and side effects of an investigational drug or treatment approach. They also look for early signs that the drug or approach is helpful.

> **Phase II trials** study how well the drug or approach works against a specific type of cancer.

> **Phase III trials** test the drug or approach against a standard treatment. If the results are good, it may be approved by the FDA.

> **Phase IV trials** study the long-term safety and benefit of an FDA-approved treatment.

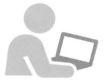

Finding a clinical trial

In the United States

NCCN Cancer Centers
NCCN.org/cancercenters

The National Cancer Institute (NCI)
cancer.gov/about-cancer/treatment/clinical-trials/search

Worldwide

The U.S. National Library of Medicine (NLM)
clinicaltrials.gov

Need help finding a clinical trial?
NCI's Cancer Information Service (CIS)
1.800.4.CANCER (1.800.422.6237)
cancer.gov/contact

Who can enroll?

Every clinical trial has rules for joining, called eligibility criteria. The rules may be about age, cancer type and stage, treatment history, or general health. These requirements ensure that participants are alike in specific ways and that the trial is as safe as possible for the participants.

Informed consent

Clinical trials are managed by a group of experts called a research team. The research team will review the study with you in detail, including its purpose and the risks and benefits of joining. All of this information is also provided in an informed consent form. Read the form carefully and ask questions before signing it. Take time to discuss with family, friends, or others whom you trust. Keep in mind that you can leave and seek treatment outside of the clinical trial at any time.

Start the conversation

Don't wait for your doctor to bring up clinical trials. Start the conversation and learn about all of your treatment options. If you find a study that you may be eligible for, ask your treatment team if you meet the requirements. If you have already started standard treatment you may not be eligible for certain clinical trials. Try not to be discouraged if you cannot join. New clinical trials are always becoming available.

Frequently asked questions

There are many myths and misconceptions surrounding clinical trials. The possible benefits and risks are not well understood by many with cancer.

Will I get a placebo?

Placebos (inactive versions of real medicines) are almost never used alone in cancer clinical trials. It is common to receive either a placebo with a standard treatment, or a new drug with a standard treatment. You will be informed, verbally and in writing, if a placebo is part of a clinical trial before you enroll.

Are clinical trials free?

There is no fee to enroll in a clinical trial. The study sponsor pays for research-related costs, including the study drug. You may, however, have costs indirectly related to the trial, such as the cost of transportation or child care due to extra appointments. During the trial, you will continue to receive standard cancer care. This care is billed to—and often covered by—insurance. You are responsible for copays and any costs for this care that are not covered by your insurance.

Supportive care

Supportive care is health care given during all cancer stages. It aims to prevent, reduce, and relieve suffering, and to improve quality of life. Supportive care might include pain relief, emotional or spiritual support, financial aid, or family counseling. Tell your care team how you are feeling and about any side effects so they can be managed. Best supportive care, supportive care, and palliative care are often used interchangeably.

It is very important to take care of yourself by eating well, drinking plenty of fluids, exercising, and doing things that make you feel energized. Strength is needed to sustain you during treatment.

Distress

Distress is an unpleasant experience of a mental, physical, social, or spiritual nature. It can affect how you feel, think, and act. Distress might include feelings of sadness, fear, helplessness, worry, anger, and guilt.

Depression, anxiety, and sleeping problems are common in cancer. Talk to your doctor and with those whom you feel most comfortable about how you are feeling. There are services and people who can help you. Support and counseling services are available.

For more information, see *NCCN Guidelines for Patients®: Distress Management – Distress During Cancer Care*, available at NCCN.org/patientguidelines.

Keep a pain diary

A pain diary is a written record that helps you keep track of when you have pain, how bad it is, what causes it, and what makes it better or worse. Use a pain diary to discuss your pain with your care team. You might be referred to a specialist for pain management.

Include in your pain diary:

- The time and dose of all medicines

- When pain starts and ends or lessens

- Where you feel pain

- Describe your pain. Is it throbbing, sharp, tingling, shooting, or burning? Is it constant, or does it come and go?

- Does the pain change at different times of day? When?

- Does the pain get worse before or after meals? Does certain food or drink make it better?

- Does the pain get better or worse with activity? What kind of activity?

- Does the pain keep you from falling asleep at night? Does pain wake you up in the night?

- Rate your pain from 0 (no pain) to 10 (worst pain you have ever felt)

- Does pain get in the way of you doing the things you enjoy?

Fatigue

Fatigue is extreme tiredness and inability to function due to lack of energy. Fatigue may be caused by cancer or it may be a side effect of treatment. Let your care team know how you are feeling and if fatigue is getting in the way of doing the things you enjoy. A balanced diet, exercise, yoga, and massage therapy can help. You might be referred to a nutritionist or dietitian to help with fatigue.

Lymphedema

Lymphedema is a condition in which extra lymph fluid builds up in tissues and causes swelling. It may occur when part of the lymph system is damaged or blocked, such as during surgery to remove lymph nodes, or radiation therapy. Swelling usually develops slowly over time. It may develop during treatment or it may start years after treatment. If you have lymphedema, you may be referred to an expert in lymphedema management. The swelling may be reduced by exercise, massage, compression sleeves, and other means. Ask your care team about the ways to treat lymphedema.

Pain

Tell your care team about any pain or discomfort. You might meet with a palliative care specialist or with a pain specialist to manage pain.

Treatment side effects

All cancer treatments can cause unwanted health issues. Such health issues are called side effects. Side effects depend on many factors. These factors include the drug type and dose, length of treatment, and the person. Some side effects may be harmful to your health. Others may just be unpleasant.

Ask for a complete list of side effects of your treatments. Also, tell your treatment team about any new or worsening symptoms. There may be ways to help you feel better. There are also ways to prevent some side effects.

Trouble eating

Sometimes side effects from surgery, cancer, or other treatments might cause you to feel not hungry or sick to your stomach (nauseated). Healthy eating is important during treatment. It includes eating a balanced diet, eating the right amount of food, and drinking enough fluids. A registered dietitian who is an expert in nutrition and food can help. Speak to your care team if you have trouble eating or maintaining your weight.

Key points

> Treatment takes a team approach. Get to know your care team and let them get to know you.

> Surgery is the main treatment for DCIS.

> Radiation therapy (RT) uses high-energy radiation from x-rays, gamma rays, protons, photons, and other sources to kill cancer cells.

> Some breast cancers grow because of estrogen. These cancers are estrogen receptor-positive (ER+) and are often treated with endocrine therapy to reduce the risk of cancer recurrence.

> A clinical trial is a type of research that studies a treatment to see how safe it is and how well it works.

> Supportive care is health care that relieves symptoms caused by treatment and improves quality of life. Supportive care is always given.

> All cancer treatments can cause unwanted health issues called side effects. It is important for you to tell your care team about all your side effects so they can be managed.

> Eating a balanced diet, drinking enough fluids, exercise, yoga, and massage therapy can help manage side effects.

It is important to tell your care team about all side effects so they can be managed.

4
Your treatment options

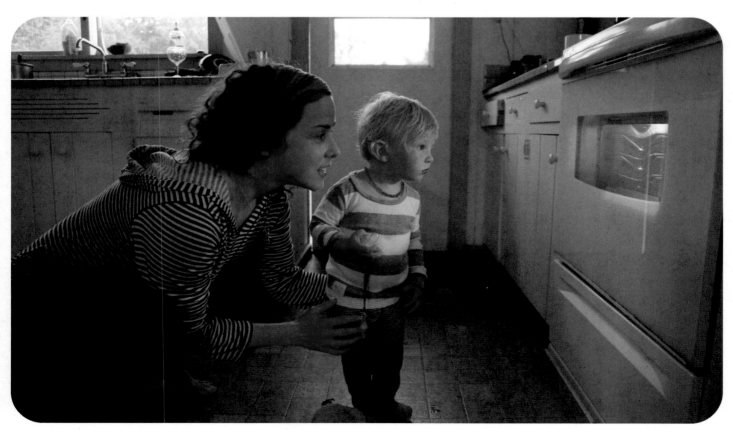

DCIS is treated with surgery. It might be surgery to remove a lump (lumpectomy) or the breast (mastectomy) with or without lymph nodes. Radiation therapy usually follows a lumpectomy. The goal of treatment is to reduce the risk of DCIS progressing to invasive breast cancer. Together, you and your doctor will choose a treatment plan that is best for you.

Overview

Ductal carcinoma in situ (DCIS) is treatable. Surgery is a central part of treatment for DCIS. Talk to your doctor about what to expect from treatment. Your preferences about treatment are important. Make your wishes known. Treatment options are found in Guide 2.

There are 2 types of treatment:

> **Local therapy** focuses on the breast and armpit (axilla) only. It includes surgery and radiation therapy.

> **Systemic therapy** works throughout the body. It includes endocrine therapy. Chemotherapy is not used to treat DCIS.

The goal of treatment is to prevent DCIS from growing outside the duct into surrounding tissue. When cancer spreads into the surrounding tissue, it is called invasive breast cancer. Invasive breast cancer is breast cancer that has spread from the milk ducts or milk glands (lobules) into the breast tissue or to nearby lymph nodes.

Guide 2 Treatment options	
Option 1	Lumpectomy with whole breast radiation therapy (WBRT)
	Lumpectomy with WBRT and radiation boost
Option 2	Lumpectomy with accelerated partial breast irradiation (APBI)
Option 3	Lumpectomy only (not an option for most people)
Option 4	Total mastectomy
	Total mastectomy with sentinel lymph node biopsy
	Flat closure or reconstruction after mastectomy

For more information on invasive breast cancer, see *NCCN Guidelines for Patients®: Breast Cancer – Invasive*, available at NCCN.org/patientguidelines.

Preventing pregnancy during treatment

If you become pregnant during radiation therapy or endocrine therapy, it can cause serious birth defects. Use birth control without hormones. Condoms are an option. Speak to your doctor about preventing pregnancy while being treated for DCIS.

Those who want to have children in the future should be referred to a fertility specialist to discuss the options before starting treatment.

Lumpectomy

A lumpectomy is also known as breast-conserving surgery (BCS). It may or may not be followed by radiation therapy. Lymph node surgery is not done with a lumpectomy.

A lumpectomy followed by radiation therapy is an option for many but not all with DCIS. This is not an option if you are pregnant, have some health issues, or the cancer is throughout the breast. The surgical margin must be cancer-free, called a negative surgical margin (R0). Lumpectomy options are described next.

Lumpectomy with whole breast radiation therapy

Most of your breast will be treated with radiation in whole breast radiation therapy (WBRT). Whole breast radiation will help to prevent the return of cancer. For every cancer that returns there is an equal chance of developing DCIS again or an invasive type of cancer. Ask your doctor if your risk of the cancer coming back is low or high. If it's high, you may receive extra radiation called a boost.

Lumpectomy with accelerated partial breast irradiation

The tumor will be removed with negative surgical margins followed by radiation therapy (RT). When RT is given only to the lumpectomy site, it is called partial breast irradiation. Accelerated partial breast irradiation (APBI) therapy is a higher dose of radiation to a smaller area, given over a shorter period of time.

Lumpectomy only

Treatment with a lumpectomy only (no radiation) is an option for a small group of people. You must have a very low risk of the cancer coming back. Surgical margins must be cancer-free. Ask your doctor if a lumpectomy without radiation is an option for you.

Mastectomy

A total mastectomy or a simple mastectomy is a surgery that removes the whole breast. Chest muscle is not removed. A skin-sparing mastectomy removes the breast but not all the skin. A nipple-sparing mastectomy preserves the nipple-areola complex (NAC) and the skin. Not everyone is a candidate for nipple-sparing mastectomy. You might choose to have a flat closure or breast reconstruction after a mastectomy.

There are many reasons why a total mastectomy might be the best choice.

> Cancer may be found at the surgical margin.

> The tumor might be large, too big, or widespread.

> You may be at risk for a second cancer.

> You might have a health issue.

> You may want a mastectomy.

> You may not be able to receive radiation to the breast area.

> Your preferences about treatment are always important. Talk to your care team and make your wishes known.

Total mastectomy with or without sentinel lymph node biopsy

The surgeon may do a sentinel lymph node biopsy (SLNB) at the time of your surgery. Sentinel lymph nodes are the first nodes cancer cells are likely to have spread. An SLNB finds and removes a few of these nodes. The nodes are then tested for cancer. Once the breast is removed, an SLNB can't be done. Instead, many lymph nodes would have to be removed to test for cancer. This is because a mastectomy permanently changes lymph flow and drainage. Therefore, if needed, an SLNB will be done at the time of a mastectomy, just in case there is a small area of invasive cancer in the breast.

Endocrine therapy after lumpectomy

Endocrine therapy is often given after a lumpectomy for cancers that are estrogen receptor-positive (ER+). This is given to reduce the risk of cancer returning. For treatment after breast-conserving surgery, see Guide 3.

Endocrine therapy

Endocrine therapy includes treatments that stop cancer growth caused by hormones. It is sometimes called hormone therapy. It is not the same as hormone replacement therapy.

If your cancer was ER+, your doctor will consider endocrine therapy. It may help reduce the risk of developing a second breast cancer in those who were treated with:

- Breast-conserving surgery (lumpectomy) with radiation therapy

- Lumpectomy alone

There is more than one type of endocrine therapy. The type prescribed by doctors is partly based on if you have menstrual periods. If you still have menstrual periods, then you are considered to be in premenopause. If your menstrual periods have stopped for more than 12 months, then you are considered to be in menopause.

- For premenopause, tamoxifen is an option.

- For menopause, tamoxifen or an aromatase inhibitor is an option. An aromatase inhibitor might be preferred if you are under 60 years of age or at risk for blood clots.

While taking endocrine therapy, you will have follow-up visits with your doctor. Tell your doctor about any side effects. There may be ways to get relief.

Guide 3
Treatment after breast-conserving surgery (lumpectomy)

Consider endocrine therapy for 5 years for those with estrogen receptor-positive (ER+) DCIS if treated with:
- Breast-conserving surgery (lumpectomy) and radiation therapy
- Lumpectomy alone

Endocrine therapy:
- For premenopause, tamoxifen
- For menopause, tamoxifen or aromatase inhibitor

Follow-up care

After treatment, you will receive follow-up care. It is important to keep any follow-up doctor visits and imaging test appointments. Contact your doctor if you have any new or worsening symptoms.

Medical history and physical exam

An update of your medical history and a physical exam are part of follow-up care. Both should be done every 6 to 12 months for 5 years. After 5 years of normal results, these tests should be done once a year.

Mammogram

A mammogram should be done every 12 months. The first one may be as soon as 6 months after a breast-conserving treatment. Mammograms aren't needed if you had both breasts removed to reduce your cancer risk.

Lowering your risk

There are things you can do to lower your chance of breast cancer in the future. Changes in your lifestyle include eating a healthy diet, exercising, limiting alcohol, and quitting smoking. You will have counseling to learn how to lower your risk.

Key points

> Ductal carcinoma in situ (DCIS) is treatable. The goal of treatment is to reduce the risk of DCIS progressing to invasive breast cancer.

> Treatment for DCIS is usually a combination of surgery and radiation therapy followed by endocrine therapy.

> Surgery options include a lumpectomy or mastectomy.

> A lumpectomy is also called breast-conserving surgery (BCS).

> A total mastectomy or a simple mastectomy is a surgery that removes the whole breast. Lymph node surgery is often done with a mastectomy.

> A skin-sparing mastectomy removes the breast but not all the skin.

> A nipple-sparing mastectomy preserves the nipple-areola complex (NAC) and the skin. Not everyone is a candidate for nipple-sparing mastectomy.

> Local therapy focuses on the breast and armpit (axilla) only. It includes surgery and radiation therapy.

> Systemic therapy works throughout the body. It includes endocrine therapy. Chemotherapy is not used to treat DCIS.

> Lifestyle changes, endocrine therapy, and surgery help to reduce the risk of future breast cancer.

> Follow-up care includes medical history, physical exams, and mammograms.

5
The breast after surgery

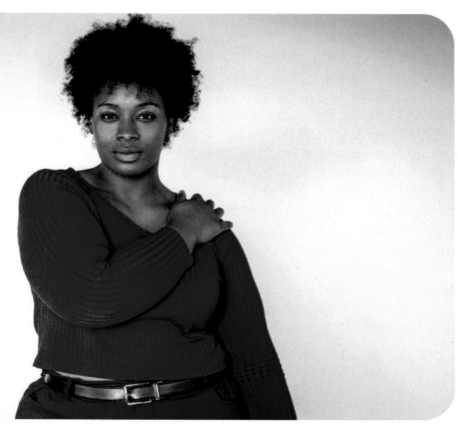

The look of your breast after surgery will depend on the type of surgery, the amount of tissue removed, and other factors such as your body type, age, and size and shape of the area before surgery. This chapter offers more information on volume displacement, flat closure, and breast reconstruction.

Volume displacement

With a lumpectomy, most people have a scar with some volume loss, but are satisfied with the way their breast looks. However, if you need a large lumpectomy and your surgeon thinks your breast will look more abnormal afterwards, your breast may be able to be re-shaped at the time of surgery. This procedure is called volume displacement or oncoplasty. It is often done by the cancer surgeon or plastic surgeon right after the lumpectomy. The surgeon will shift the remaining breast tissue to fill the gap left by the removed tumor.

If volume displacement is planned, a larger piece of your breast will need to be removed. Despite a larger piece being removed, the natural look of your breast will be kept.

You may not like the results of the volume displacement. In this case, breast revision surgery may help. This surgery is done by a plastic surgeon. A second volume displacement may be an option, too. Another option is to get breast implants or mastectomy with reconstruction.

Flat closure

In a total mastectomy with a flat closure, the entire breast, including nipple, extra skin, fat, and other tissue in the breast area are removed. The remaining skin is tightened and sewn together. No breast mound is created and no implant is added. The scar will be slightly raised and differ in color than the surrounding skin. A flat closure is not completely flat or smooth. The end result varies from person to person. Ask to look at "after" pictures from flat closures so you know what to expect.

You might decide to have a flat closure procedure at a later time or after having breast implants removed. Talk to your care team to learn more.

Breast reconstruction

Breast reconstruction is surgery to rebuild the shape and look of the breast after a mastectomy. In many cases, breast reconstruction involves a staged approach. It might require more than one procedure.

You may have a choice as to when breast reconstruction is done. Immediate reconstruction is finished within hours after removing the breast. Delayed reconstruction can occur months or years after the cancer surgery. Reconstruction can also be done in a staged fashion, with part of the reconstruction done at the time of the original cancer surgery, and finished with another surgery at a later time. A plastic surgeon performs breast reconstruction.

Breasts can be reconstructed with implants and flaps. All methods are generally safe, but as with any surgery, there are risks. Ask your treatment team for a complete list of side effects.

Implants

Breast implants are small bags filled with salt water, silicone gel, or both. They are placed under the breast skin or muscle to look like a new breast following a mastectomy. A balloon-like device, called an expander, may be used first to stretch out tissue. It will be placed under your skin or muscle and enlarged every few weeks for two to three months. When your skin is stretched to the proper size, you will have surgery to place the final implant.

Implants have a small risk of leaking or causing other issues. You may feel pain from the implant or expander. Scar tissue or tissue death can occur. Textured implants can cause breast implant-associated anaplastic large cell lymphoma (BIA-ALCL), a type of cancer.

Flaps

Sometimes breast fullness can be recreated after a skin-sparing mastectomy. In a skin-sparing mastectomy, breast tissue is removed from underneath the skin. The nipple remains intact, if possible. The remaining skin flaps are used to create a breast mound. This technique does not use implants or skin transferred from other parts of the body and may be completed in a single surgery. This is best suited for those with larger breasts who are willing to have much smaller breasts as a result.

Breasts can be remade using tissue from other parts of your body, known as "flaps." These flaps are taken from the abdomen, buttocks, thigh, or from under the shoulder blade. Some flaps are completely removed and then sewn in place. Other flaps stay attached to your body but are slid over and sewn into place.

There are several risks associated with flaps, including death of fat in the flap, which can cause lumps. A hernia may result from muscle weakness. Problems are more likely to occur among those who have diabetes or who smoke.

Implants and flaps

Some breasts are reconstructed with both implants and flaps. This method may give the reconstructed breast more volume to match the other breast. For any reconstruction, you may need surgery on your remaining breast to match the two breasts in size and shape.

Nipple replacement

Like your breast, a nipple can be remade. To rebuild a nipple, a plastic surgeon can use surrounding tissues. Also, nipples can be remade with tissue from the thigh, other nipple, or the sex organs between your legs (vulva). Tissue can be darkened with a tattoo to look more like a nipple. It is important to note that while you can remake something to look like a nipple, it will not have the sensation of your real nipple. Also, a tattoo can be done to look like a nipple without having to take tissue from another part of the body.

What to consider

Some things to consider when deciding to have flat closure or reconstruction after mastectomy:

> **Your desire** - You may have a strong feeling towards flat closure or one form of reconstruction after being given the options. Breast reconstruction should be a shared decision between you and your care team. Make your wishes known.

> **Health issues** - You may have health issues such as diabetes or a blood disorder that might affect or delay healing, or make longer procedures unsafe.

> **Tobacco use** - Smoking delays wound healing and can cause mastectomy flap death (necrosis), nipple-areola complex (NAC) necrosis in a nipple-sparing mastectomy, infection, and failure of implant-based reconstruction. In free flap reconstruction, smoking increases the risk of complications. You are encouraged to stop smoking prior to reconstruction.

> **Breast size and shape** – There are limits to the available sizes of breast implants. Very large breasts or breasts that lack tone or droop (called ptosis) might be difficult to match. Breast reduction surgery might be an option.

> **Body mass index (BMI)** – Those with an elevated BMI have increased risk of infections and complications with breast reconstruction.

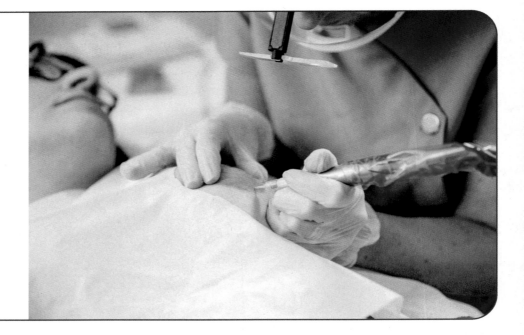

Tattoo

Removed nipples can be remade with body tissue and/or tattooing.

Key points

- Volume displacement is a shifting of the breast tissue to fill the gap left by a lumpectomy.

- Flat closure is done after a mastectomy in which the skin is tightened and sewn together without the addition of a breast implant.

- Breast reconstruction is surgery to rebuild the shape and look of the breast.

- Breasts that are fully removed in a mastectomy can be remade with breast implants, flaps, or both.

- Removed nipples can be remade with body tissue and/or tattooing.

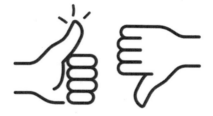

Let us know what you think!

Please take a moment to complete an online survey about the NCCN Guidelines for Patients.

NCCN.org/patients/response

6
Making treatment decisions

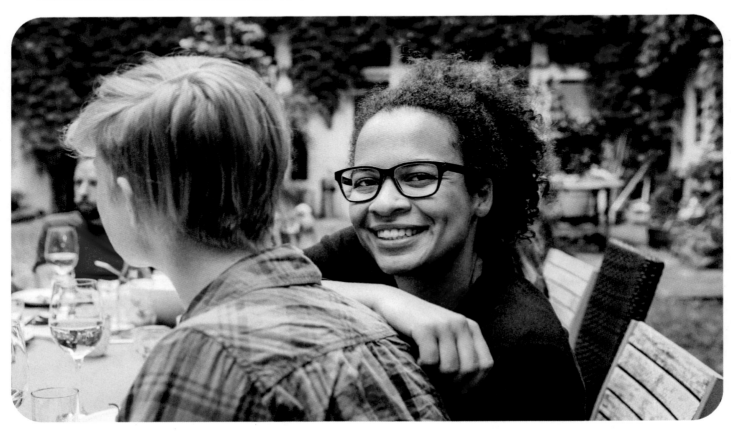

It's important to be comfortable with the cancer treatment you choose. This choice starts with having an open and honest conversation with your doctor.

It's your choice

In shared decision-making, you and your doctors share information, discuss the options, and agree on a treatment plan. It starts with an open and honest conversation between you and your doctor.

Treatment decisions are very personal. What is important to you may not be important to someone else.

Some things that may play a role in your decision-making:

> What you want and how that might differ from what others want

> Your religious and spiritual beliefs

> Your feelings about certain treatments like surgery or endocrine therpay

> Your feelings about pain or side effects

> Cost of treatment, travel to treatment centers, and time away from school or work

> Quality of life and length of life

> How active you are and the activities that are important to you

Think about what you want from treatment. Discuss openly the risks and benefits of specific treatments and procedures. Weigh options and share concerns with your doctor.

If you take the time to build a relationship with your doctor, it will help you feel supported when considering options and making treatment decisions.

Second opinion
It is normal to want to start treatment as soon as possible. While cancer can't be ignored, there is time to have another doctor review your test results and suggest a treatment plan. This is called getting a second opinion, and it's a normal part of cancer care. Even doctors get second opinions!

Things you can do to prepare:

> Check with your insurance company about its rules on second opinions. There may be out-of-pocket costs to see doctors who are not part of your insurance plan.

> Make plans to have copies of all your records sent to the doctor you will see for your second opinion.

Support groups
Many people diagnosed with cancer find support groups to be helpful. Support groups often include people at different stages of treatment. Some people may be newly diagnosed, while others may be finished with treatment. If your hospital or community doesn't have support groups for people with cancer, check out the websites listed in this book.

Questions to ask your doctors

Possible questions to ask your doctors are listed on the following pages. Feel free to use these questions or come up with your own. Be clear about your goals for treatment and find out what to expect from treatment.

Questions to ask about testing and diagnosis

1. What tests will I have? How often will they be repeated? Will my insurance pay for these tests?

2. What will you do to make me comfortable during testing?

3. What if I am pregnant or want to become pregnant?

4. When will I have a biopsy? Will I have more than one? What are the risks?

5. How will my biopsy be performed? What else might be done at this time?

6. How soon will I know the results and who will explain them to me?

7. How can I get a copy of the pathology report and other test results?

8. Who will talk with me about the next steps? When?

9. What can I do before my next appointment?

Questions to ask your care team about their experience

1. What is your experience treating DCIS?

2. What is the experience of those on your team?

3. Do you only treat DCIS? What else do you treat?

4. How many patients like me (of the same age, gender, race) have you treated?

5. Will you be consulting with experts to discuss my care? Whom will you consult?

6. How many procedures like the one you're suggesting have you done?

7. Is this treatment a major part of your practice?

8. How many of your patients have had complications? What were the complications?

9. How many breast cancer surgeries have you done? What type of surgeries have you done? How many per year?

10. Who will manage my day-to-day care?

Questions to ask about options

1. What will happen if I do nothing?

2. How do my age, overall health, and other factors affect my options?

3. What if I am pregnant? What if I'm planning to get pregnant in the near future?

4. Which option is proven to work best for my cancer, age, and other risk factors?

5. What are the possible complications and side effects?

6. How do you know if the treatment worked? How will I know?

7. What can be done to prevent or relieve the side effects of treatment?

8. Are there any life-threatening side effects of this treatment? How will I be monitored?

9. Am I a candidate for a clinical trial? Can I join a clinical trial at any time?

10. Does any option offer a long-term cancer control? Are the chances any better for one option than another? Less time-consuming? Less expensive?

11. Is there a social worker or someone who can help me decide?

12. Is there a hospital or treatment center you can recommend for breast cancer treatment? Can I go to one hospital for surgery and a different center for radiation therapy?

Questions to ask about treatment

1. What are my treatment choices? What are the benefits and risks? Which treatment do you recommend and why?

2. How will my age, performance status, cancer stage, and other health conditions limit my treatment choices?

3. Does the order of treatment matter?

4. How long do I have to decide about treatment?

5. Will I have to go to the hospital or elsewhere for treatment? How often? How long is each visit? Will I have to stay overnight in the hospital or make travel plans?

6. Do I have a choice of when to begin treatment? Can I choose the days and times of treatment? Should I bring someone with me?

7. How much will the treatment hurt? What will you do to make me comfortable?

8. Can I stop treatment at any time? What will happen if I stop treatment?

9. How much will this treatment cost me? How much will my insurance pay for this treatment? Are there any programs to help me pay for treatment?

10. Will I miss work or school? Will I be able to drive? When will I be able to return to my normal activities?

11. What are the chances my cancer will return after this treatment? How will it be treated if it returns?

12. I would like a second opinion. Is there someone you can recommend? Who can help me gather all of my records for a second opinion?

Questions to ask about surgery

1. How much of my breast will be removed? What will it look like afterwards?

2. What lymph nodes might be removed during surgery? What will this mean in terms of my recovery?

3. What kind of surgery will I have? Will I have more than one surgery?

4. What are the chances you can remove the whole tumor and I will have a negative margin?

5. How long will it take me to recover from surgery? When will I be able to return to work?

6. How much pain will I be in? What will be done to manage my pain?

7. What is the chance that this surgery will shorten my life?

8. What other side effects can I expect from surgery? What complications can occur from this surgery?

9. What treatment will I have before, during, or after surgery? What does this treatment do?

10. I am considering a mastectomy with flat closure. Can you tell me more about this procedure?

11. I am considering a mastectomy with reconstruction. Can you tell me about the options?

Questions to ask about radiation therapy

1. What type of radiation therapy (RT) will I have?

2. What will you target?

3. What is the goal of this RT?

4. How many treatment sessions will I require? Can you do a shorter course of RT?

5. Do you offer this type of RT here? If not, can you refer me to someone who does?

6. What side effects can I expect from RT?

7. Should I eat or drink before RT?

8. Will I be given medicine to help me relax during RT?

9. What should I wear?

Questions to ask about side effects

1. What are the side effects of treatment?

2. How long will these side effects last? Do any side effects lessen or worsen in severity over time?

3. What side effects should I watch for? What side effects are expected and which are life threatening?

4. When should I call the doctor? Can I text? What should I do on weekends and during non-office hours?

5. What emergency department or ER should I go to? Will my treatment team be able to communicate with the ER team?

6. What medicines can I take to prevent or relieve side effects?

7. What can I do to help with pain and other side effects?

8. Will you stop treatment or change treatment if there are side effects? What do you look for?

9. What can I do to lessen or prevent side effects? What will you do?

10. What medicines may worsen side effects of treatment?

Questions to ask about clinical trials

1. What clinical trials are available for my type and stage of breast cancer?

2. What are the treatments used in the clinical trial?

3. What does the treatment do?

4. Has the treatment been used before? Has it been used for other types of cancer?

5. What are the risks and benefits of this treatment?

6. What side effects should I expect? How will the side effects be controlled?

7. How long will I be in the clinical trial?

8. Will I be able to get other treatments if this doesn't work?

9. How will you know the treatment is working?

10. Will the clinical trial cost me anything? If so, how much?

11. How do I find out about clinical trials that I can participate in? Are there online sources that I can search?

Resources

American Association for Cancer Research (AACR)
aacr.org/

American Breast Cancer Foundation
youandbreastcancer.com/en-bc/home

American Cancer Society (ACS)
cancer.org/cancer/breast-cancer.html

Breast Cancer Alliance (BCA)
breastcanceralliance.org

Breast Cancer Support Project
breastcancerportraitproject.org

Breastcancer.org
breastcancer.org

Brem Foundation
bremfoundation.org

CancerCare
cancercare.org

Cancer Support Community
cancersupportcommunity.org/living-cancer

Chemocare
chemocare.com

DiepCFoundation
diepcfoundation.org

FORCE - Facing Our Risk of Cancer Empowered
facingourrisk.org

GPAC - Global Patient Advocacy Coalition
GPACunited.org

Living Beyond Breast Cancer (LBBC)
lbbc.org

MedlinePlus
medlineplus.gov/breastcancer.html

My Survival Story
mysurvivalstory.org

National Cancer Institute (NCI)
cancer.gov/types/breast

National Center for Health Research
breastimplantinfo.org

National Coalition for Cancer Survivorship
canceradvocacy.org/toolbox

National Financial Resource Directory - Patient Advocate Foundation
patientadvocate.org/explore-our-resources/national-financial-resource-directory/

OncoLink
oncolink.org

Patient Access Network Foundation
panfoundation.org

Radiological Society of North America
radiologyinfo.org

SHARE Cancer Support
sharecancersupport.org

Sharsheret
sharsheret.org

Smart Patients
smartpatients.com/communities/breast-cancer

Susan G. Komen
komen.org

Testing.com
testing.com

The Male Breast Cancer Coalition
malebreastcancercoalition.org/men-have-breasts-too

Unite for HER
uniteforher.org

Young Survival Coalition (YSC)
youngsurvival.org

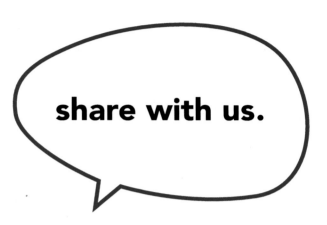

Take our <u>survey</u>
**And help make the
NCCN Guidelines for Patients
better for everyone!**

NCCN.org/patients/comments

Words to know

accelerated partial breast irradiation (APBI)
Treatment with radiation of part of the breast with cancer. A higher dose is given over a shorter period of time compared to whole breast radiation therapy.

areola
A darker, round area of skin on the breast around the nipple.

aromatase inhibitor (AI)
A drug that lowers the level of estrogen in the body.

bilateral diagnostic mammogram
Pictures of the insides of both breasts that are made from a set of x-rays.

biopsy
A procedure that removes fluid or tissue samples to be tested for a disease.

boost
An extra dose of radiation to a specific area of the body.

breast-conserving surgery (BCS)
A cancer treatment that includes removing a breast lump.

breast implant
A small bag filled with salt water, gel, or both that is used to remake breasts.

breast reconstruction
An operation that creates new breasts.

cancer stage
A rating of the outlook of a cancer based on its growth and spread.

carcinoma
A cancer of cells that line the inner or outer surfaces of the body.

chest wall
The layer of muscle, bone, and fat that protects the vital organs.

clinical breast exam
Touching of a breast by a health expert to feel for diseases.

clinical stage (c)
The rating of the extent of cancer before treatment is started.

clinical trial
A type of research that assesses health tests or treatments.

connective tissue
Supporting and binding tissue that surrounds other tissues and organs.

contrast
A substance put into your body to make clearer pictures during imaging tests.

core needle biopsy
A procedure that removes tissue samples with a hollow needle. Also called core biopsy.

diagnostic bilateral mammogram
Pictures of the insides of both breasts that are made from a set of x-rays.

duct
A tube-shaped structure through which milk travels to the nipple.

ductal carcinoma in situ (DCIS)
A breast cancer that has not grown outside the breast ducts.

endocrine therapy
A cancer treatment that stops the making or action of estrogen. Also called hormone therapy.

estrogen
A hormone that causes female body traits.

estrogen receptor (ER)
A protein inside cells that binds to estrogen.

estrogen receptor-negative (ER-)
A type of breast cancer that doesn't use estrogen to grow.

estrogen receptor-positive (ER+)
A type of breast cancer that uses estrogen to grow.

fertility specialist
An expert who helps people to have babies.

fine-needle aspiration (FNA)
A procedure that removes tissue samples with a very thin needle.

flat closure
Procedure done after a mastectomy in which the skin is tightened and sewn together without the addition of a breast implant.

gene
Coded instructions in cells for making new cells and controlling how cells behave.

genetic counseling
Expert guidance on the chance for a disease that is passed down in families.

hereditary breast cancer
Breast cancer that was likely caused by abnormal genes passed down from parent to child.

histology
The structure of cells, tissue, and organs as viewed under a microscope.

hormone
A chemical in the body that triggers a response from cells or organs.

immunohistochemistry (IHC)
A lab test of cancer cells to find specific cell traits involved in abnormal cell growth.

invasive breast cancer
The growth of breast cancer into the breast's supporting tissue (stroma).

lobule
A gland in the breast that makes breast milk.

lobular carcinoma in situ (LCIS)
A benign (non-cancerous) condition in which abnormal cells are found in the lobules of the breast.

lumpectomy
An operation that removes a small breast cancer tumor. Also called breast-conserving surgery.

lymph
A clear fluid containing white blood cells.

lymph node
A small, bean-shaped disease-fighting structure.

lymphadenopathy
Lymph nodes that are abnormal in size or consistency.

lymphatic system
Germ-fighting network of tissues and organs that includes the bone marrow, spleen, thymus, lymph nodes, and lymphatic vessels. Part of the immune system.

lymphedema
Swelling in the body due to a buildup of fluid called lymph.

magnetic resonance imaging (MRI)
A test that uses radio waves and powerful magnets to make pictures of the insides of the body.

mammogram
A picture of the insides of the breast that is made by an x-ray test.

mastectomy
An operation that removes the whole breast.

medical history
A report of all your health events and medications.

medical oncologist
A doctor who is an expert in cancer drugs.

menopause
The point in time 12 months after a last menstrual period.

mutation
An abnormal change.

nipple-areola complex (NAC)
The ring of darker breast skin is called the areola. The raised tip within the areola is called the nipple.

noninvasive breast cancer
Breast cancer that has not grown into tissue from which it can spread.

palpable adenopathy
Lymph nodes that feel abnormal in size or consistency.

partial breast irradiation
Treatment with radiation that is received at the site of the removed breast tumor.

pathologic stage (p)
A rating of the extent of cancer based on tests given after treatment.

pathologist
A doctor who's an expert in testing cells and tissue to find disease.

postmenopause
The state of having no more menstrual periods.

premenopause
The state of having menstrual periods.

primary tumor
The first mass of cancer cells.

prognosis
The likely course and outcome of a disease based on tests.

radiation therapy (RT)
A treatment that uses high-energy rays.

recurrence
The return of cancer after a cancer-free period.

sentinel lymph node (SLN)
The first lymph node to which cancer cells spread after leaving a tumor.

sentinel lymph node biopsy (SLNB)
An operation to remove the disease-fighting structures (lymph nodes) to which cancer first spreads. Also called sentinel lymph node dissection.

side effect
An unhealthy or unpleasant physical or emotional response to treatment.

skin-sparing mastectomy
An operation that removes all breast tissue but saves as much breast skin as possible.

supportive care
Health care that includes symptom relief but not cancer treatment. Also called palliative care or best supportive care.

surgical margin
The normal-looking tissue around a tumor that was removed during an operation.

systemic therapy
Drug treatment that works throughout the body.

total mastectomy
An operation that removes the entire breast but no chest muscles. Also called simple mastectomy.

ultrasound
A test that uses sound waves to take pictures of the inside of the body.

vulva
The outer female organs that are between the legs.

volume displacement
A method to shift breast tissue during an operation to fill a gap.

whole breast radiation therapy (WBRT)
Treatment with radiation of the entire breast.

NCCN Contributors

This patient guide is based on the NCCN Clinical Practice Guidelines in Oncology (NCCN Guidelines®) for Breast Cancer, Version 2.2022. It was adapted, reviewed, and published with help from the following people:

Dorothy A. Shead, MS
Senior Director
Patient Information Operations

Tanya Fischer, MEd, MSLIS
Medical Writer

Susan Kidney
Senior Graphic Design Specialist

The NCCN Clinical Practice Guidelines in Oncology (NCCN Guidelines®) for Breast Cancer, Version 2.2022 were developed by the following NCCN Panel Members:

William J. Gradishar, MD/Chair
Robert H. Lurie Comprehensive Cancer Center of Northwestern University

Meena S. Moran, MD/Vice-Chair
Yale Cancer Center/Smilow Cancer Hospital

Jame Abraham, MD
Case Comprehensive Cancer Center/ University Hospitals Seidman Cancer Center and Cleveland Clinic Taussig Cancer Institute

*Rebecca Aft, MD, PhD
Siteman Cancer Center at Barnes-Jewish Hospital and Washington University School of Medicine

Doreen Agnese, MD
The Ohio State University Comprehensive Cancer Center - James Cancer Hospital and Solove Research Institute

Kimberly H. Allison, MD
Stanford Cancer Institute

*Bethany Anderson, MD
University of Wisconsin Carbone Cancer Center

Sarah L. Blair, MD
UC San Diego Moores Cancer Center

Harold J. Burstein, MD, PhD
Dana-Farber/Brigham and Women's Cancer Center

Helen Chew, MD
UC Davis Comprehensive Cancer Center

Chau Dang, MD
Memorial Sloan Kettering Cancer Center

Anthony D. Elias, MD
University of Colorado Cancer Center

Sharon H. Giordano, MD, MPH
The University of Texas MD Anderson Cancer Center

Matthew Goetz, MD
Mayo Clinic Cancer Center

Lori J. Goldstein, MD
Fox Chase Cancer Center

Sara A. Hurvitz, MD
UCLA Jonsson Comprehensive Cancer Center

Steven J. Isakoff, MD, PhD
Massachusetts General Hospital Cancer Center

Rachel C. Jankowitz, MD
Abramson Cancer Center at the University of Pennsylvania

*Sara H. Javid, MD
Fred Hutchinson Cancer Research Center/Seattle Cancer Care Alliance

Jairam Krishnamurthy, MD
Fred & Pamela Buffet Cancer Center

Marilyn Leitch, MD
UT Southwestern Simmons Comprehensive Cancer Center

*Janice Lyons, MD
Case Comprehensive Cancer Center/ University Hospitals Seidman Cancer Center and Cleveland Clinic Taussig Cancer Institute

Ingrid A. Mayer, MD
Vanderbilt-Ingram Cancer Center

Joanne Mortimer, MD
City of Hope National Medical Center

Sameer A. Patel, MD
Fox Chase Cancer Center

Lori J. Pierce, MD
University of Michigan Rogel Cancer Center

Laura H. Rosenberger, MD, MS
Duke Cancer Institute

Hope S. Rugo, MD
UCSF Helen Diller Family Comprehensive Cancer Center

Amy Sitapati, MD
UC San Diego Moores Cancer Center

Karen Lisa Smith, MD, MPH
The Sidney Kimmel Comprehensive Cancer Center at Johns Hopkins

*Mary Lou Smith, JD, MBA
Patient Advocate
Research Advocacy Network

Hatem Soliman, MD
Moffitt Cancer Center

Erica M. Stringer-Reasor, MD
O'Neal Comprehensive Cancer Center at UAB

Melinda L. Telli, MD
Stanford Cancer Institute

John H. Ward, MD
Huntsman Cancer Institute at the University of Utah

Kari B. Wisinski, MD
University of Wisconsin Carbone Cancer Center

Jessica S. Young, MD
Roswell Park Comprehensive Cancer Center

NCCN Staff

Rashmi Kumar, PhD
Director, Clinical Information Operations

Jennifer Burns, BS
Manager, Guidelines Supportion

* Reviewed this patient guide. For disclosures, visit NCCN.org/disclosures.

NCCN Cancer Centers

Abramson Cancer Center
at the University of Pennsylvania
Philadelphia, Pennsylvania
800.789.7366 • pennmedicine.org/cancer

Case Comprehensive Cancer Center/
University Hospitals Seidman Cancer
Center and Cleveland Clinic Taussig
Cancer Institute
Cleveland, Ohio
800.641.2422 • UH Seidman Cancer Center
uhhospitals.org/services/cancer-services
866.223.8100 • CC Taussig Cancer Institute
my.clevelandclinic.org/departments/cancer
216.844.8797 • Case CCC
case.edu/cancer

City of Hope National Medical Center
Los Angeles, California
800.826.4673 • cityofhope.org

Dana-Farber/Brigham and Women's
Cancer Center | Massachusetts General
Hospital Cancer Center
Boston, Massachusetts
617.732.5500 • youhaveus.org
617.726.5130
massgeneral.org/cancer-center

Duke Cancer Institute
Durham, North Carolina
888.275.3853 • dukecancerinstitute.org

Fox Chase Cancer Center
Philadelphia, Pennsylvania
888.369.2427 • foxchase.org

Fred & Pamela Buffett Cancer Center
Omaha, Nebraska
402.559.5600 • unmc.edu/cancercenter

Fred Hutchinson Cancer
Research Center/Seattle
Cancer Care Alliance
Seattle, Washington
206.606.7222 • seattlecca.org
206.667.5000 • fredhutch.org

Huntsman Cancer Institute
at the University of Utah
Salt Lake City, Utah
800.824.2073 • huntsmancancer.org

Indiana University
Melvin and Bren Simon
Comprehensive Cancer Center
Indianapolis, Indiana
www.cancer.iu.edu

Mayo Clinic Cancer Center
Phoenix/Scottsdale, Arizona
Jacksonville, Florida
Rochester, Minnesota
480.301.8000 • Arizona
904.953.0853 • Florida
507.538.3270 • Minnesota
mayoclinic.org/cancercenter

Memorial Sloan Kettering
Cancer Center
New York, New York
800.525.2225 • mskcc.org

Moffitt Cancer Center
Tampa, Florida
888.663.3488 • moffitt.org

O'Neal Comprehensive
Cancer Center at UAB
Birmingham, Alabama
800.822.0933 • uab.edu/onealcancercenter

Robert H. Lurie Comprehensive Cancer
Center of Northwestern University
Chicago, Illinois
866.587.4322 • cancer.northwestern.edu

Roswell Park Comprehensive
Cancer Center
Buffalo, New York
877.275.7724 • roswellpark.org

Siteman Cancer Center at Barnes-
Jewish Hospital and Washington
University School of Medicine
St. Louis, Missouri
800.600.3606 • siteman.wustl.edu

St. Jude Children's
Research Hospital/
The University of Tennessee
Health Science Center
Memphis, Tennessee
866.278.5833 • stjude.org
901.448.5500 • uthsc.edu

Stanford Cancer Institute
Stanford, California
877.668.7535 • cancer.stanford.edu

The Ohio State University
Comprehensive Cancer Center -
James Cancer Hospital and
Solove Research Institute
Columbus, Ohio
800.293.5066 • cancer.osu.edu

The Sidney Kimmel Comprehensive
Cancer Center at Johns Hopkins
Baltimore, Maryland
410.955.8964
www.hopkinskimmelcancercenter.org

The University of Texas
MD Anderson Cancer Center
Houston, Texas
844.269.5922 • mdanderson.org

UC Davis
Comprehensive Cancer Center
Sacramento, California
916.734.5959 • 800.770.9261
health.ucdavis.edu/cancer

UC San Diego Moores Cancer Center
La Jolla, California
858.822.6100 • cancer.ucsd.edu

UCLA Jonsson
Comprehensive Cancer Center
Los Angeles, California
310.825.5268 • cancer.ucla.edu

UCSF Helen Diller Family
Comprehensive Cancer Center
San Francisco, California
800.689.8273 • cancer.ucsf.edu

University of Colorado Cancer Center
Aurora, Colorado
720.848.0300 • coloradocancercenter.org

University of Michigan
Rogel Cancer Center
Ann Arbor, Michigan
800.865.1125 • rogelcancercenter.org

University of Wisconsin
Carbone Cancer Center
Madison, Wisconsin
608.265.1700 • uwhealth.org/cancer

UT Southwestern Simmons
Comprehensive Cancer Center
Dallas, Texas
214.648.3111 • utsouthwestern.edu/simmons

Vanderbilt-Ingram Cancer Center
Nashville, Tennessee
877.936.8422 • vicc.org

Yale Cancer Center/
Smilow Cancer Hospital
New Haven, Connecticut
855.4.SMILOW • yalecancercenter.org

Notes

Index

Made in the USA
Monee, IL
07 January 2023

24730772R00040